Look out

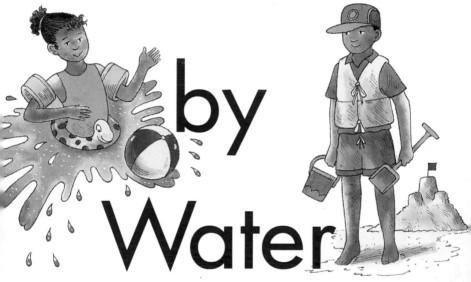

by

Water

Helena Ramsay

Illustrated by

Colin King

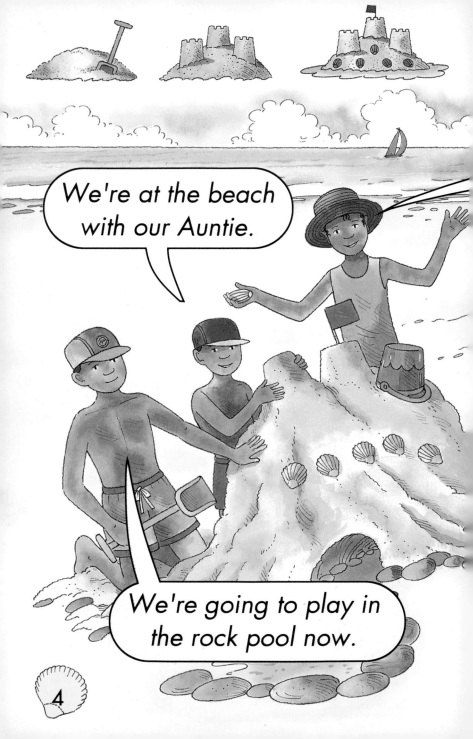

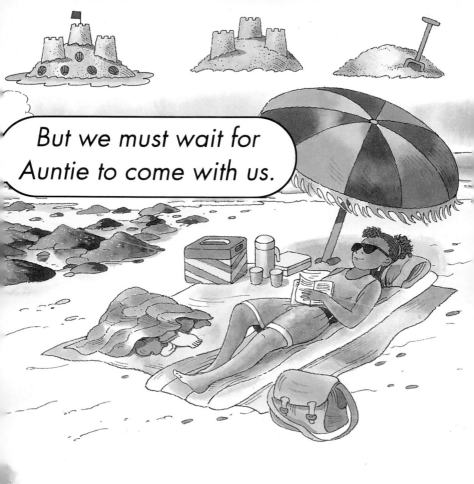

You must always have a grown-up with you when you are near water.
Never go on your own.

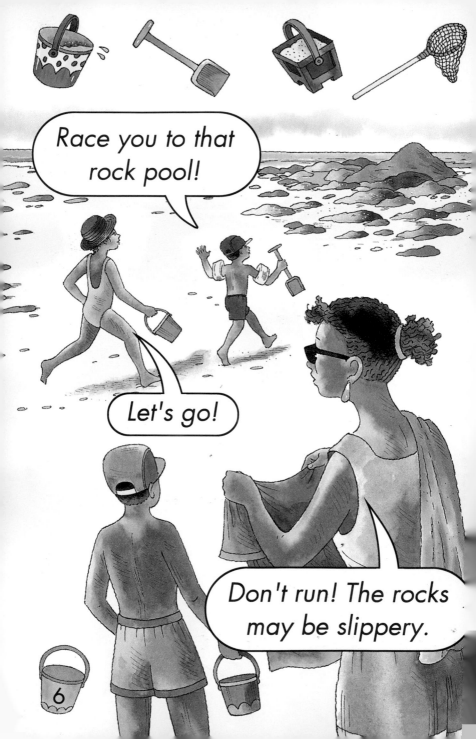

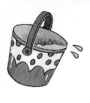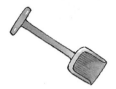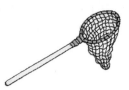

The ground is often slippery near water. If you run, you might fall over and hurt yourself.

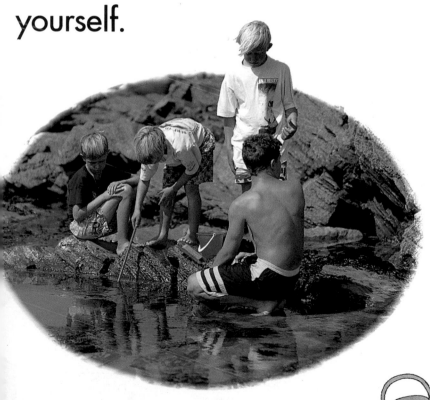

7

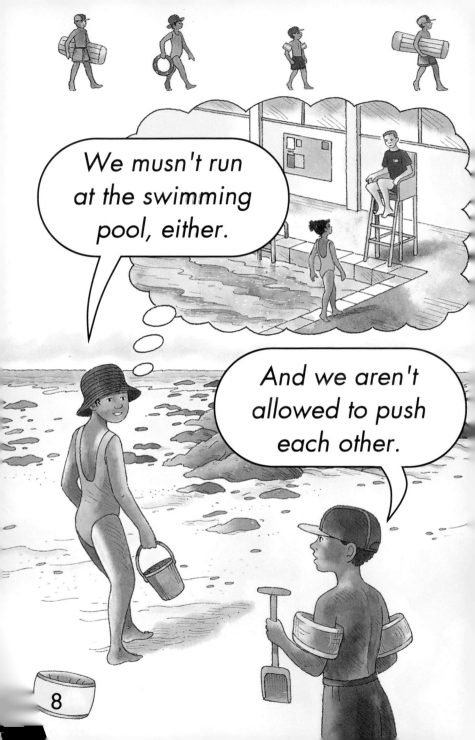

8

Never behave in a silly way
when you are near water.
There might be
an accident.

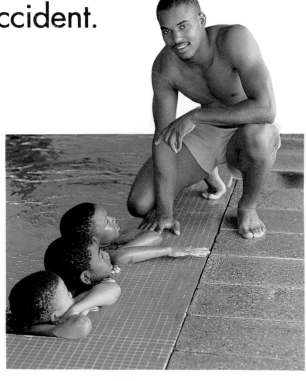

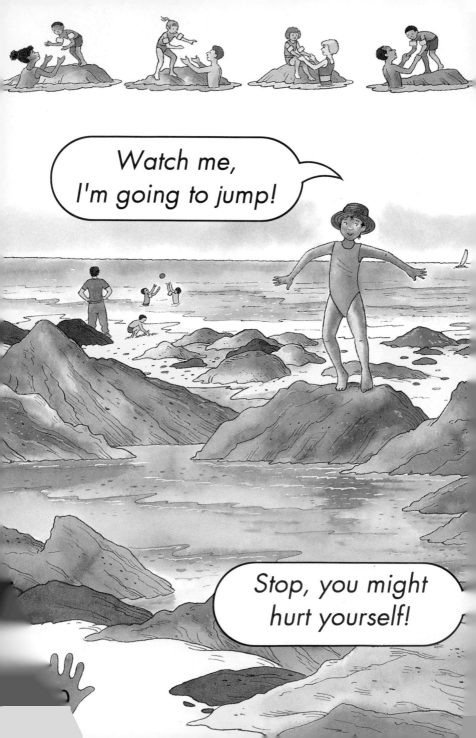

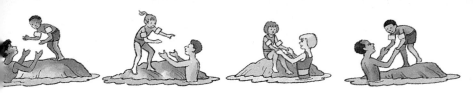

Never jump or dive into water unless you know how deep it is.

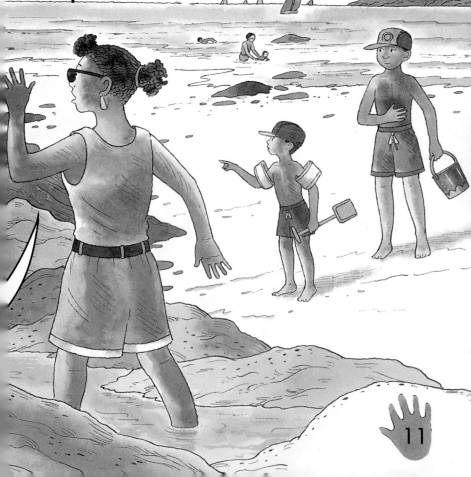

11

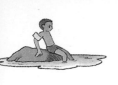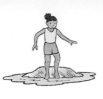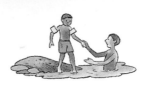

Always find a safe place to get in and out of the water.

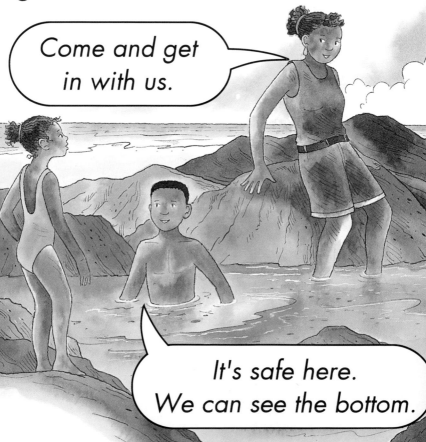

12

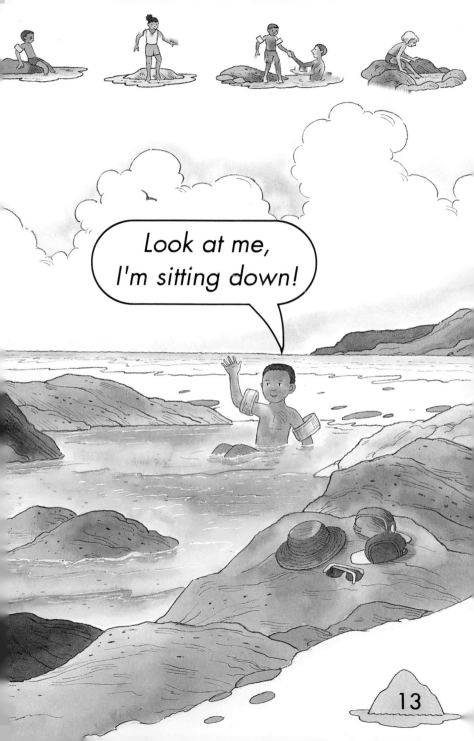

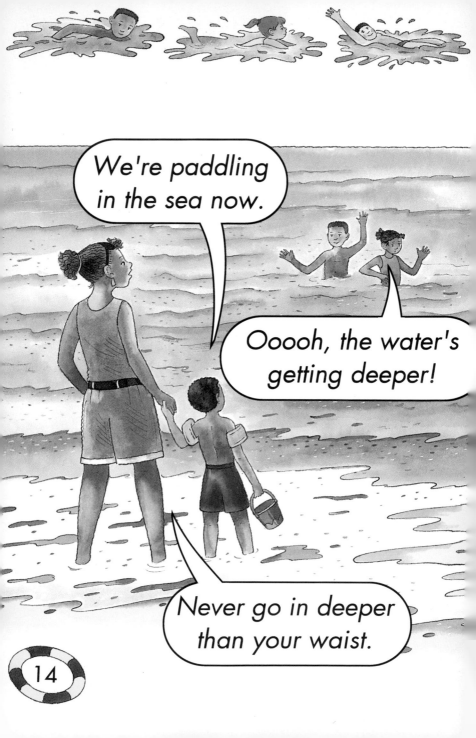

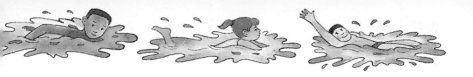

The water can get deeper
very suddenly at the seaside.
Be careful never to get out
of your depth.

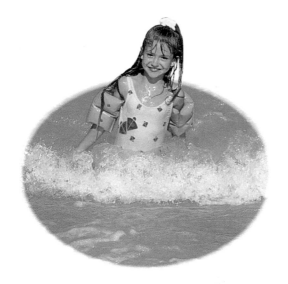

15

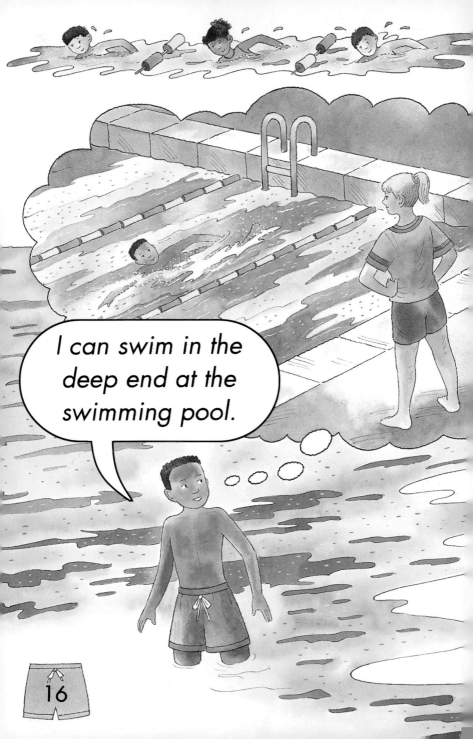

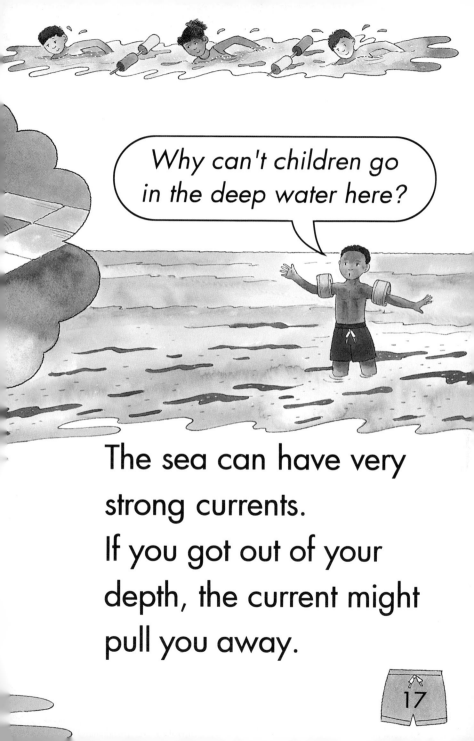

Why can't children go in the deep water here?

The sea can have very strong currents.
If you got out of your depth, the current might pull you away.

17

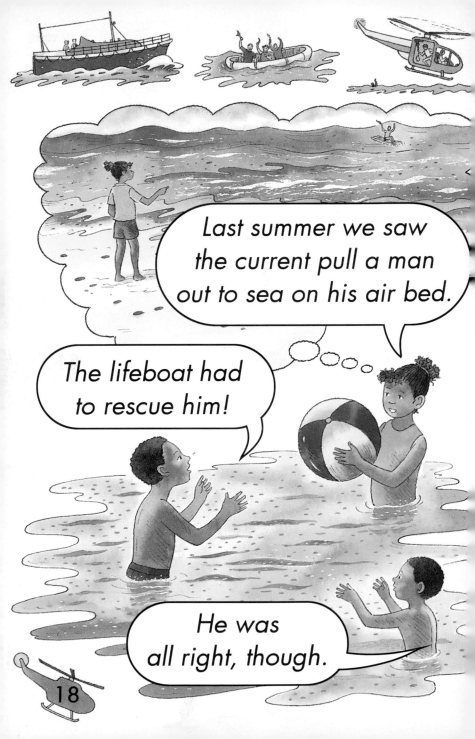

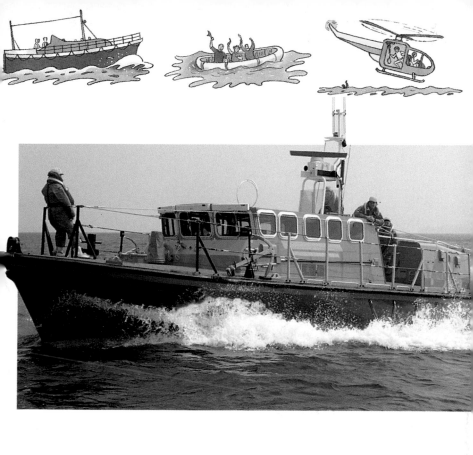

It's dangerous to play on air beds at the seaside. You might be pulled out to sea by the current.

19

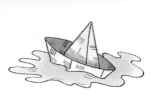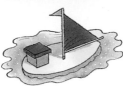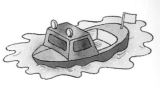

There's a strong current in the river at home, too.

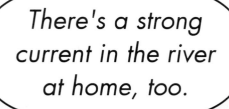

When we throw sticks into the water it carries them away.

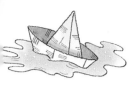 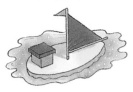 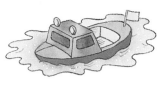

Never swim in rivers and lakes, it's too dangerous.

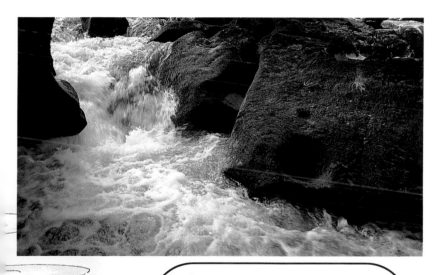

The current carried my toy boat away.

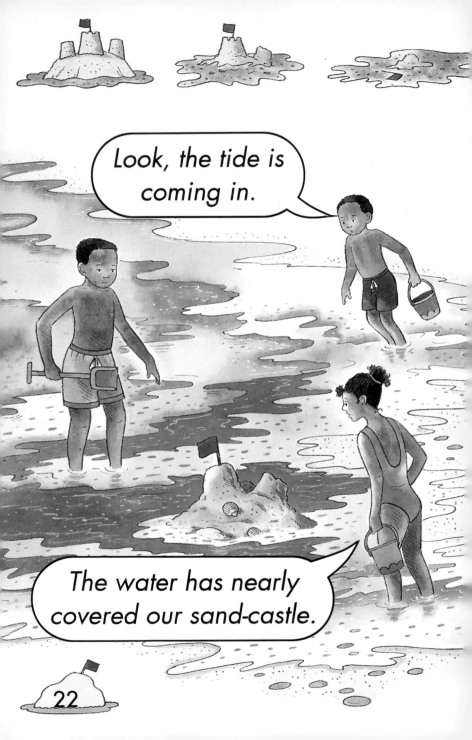

22

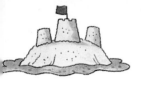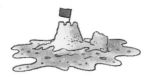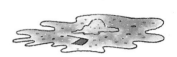

The tide can come in very quickly.

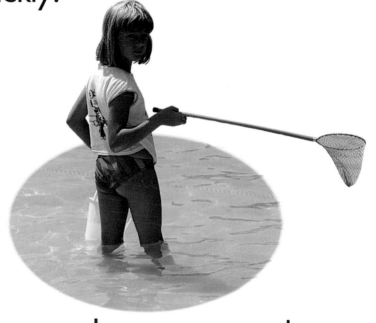

Always take care not to be cut off from the beach by deep water.

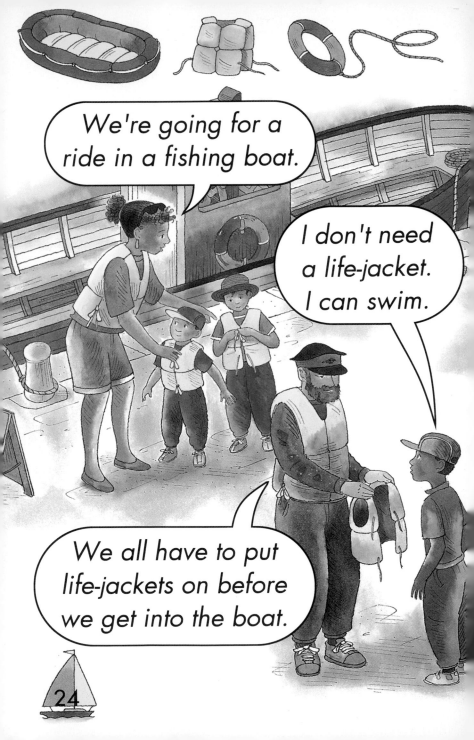

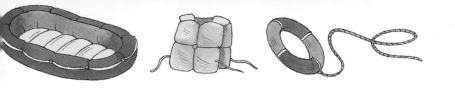

Everybody should wear a
life-jacket when they go
on a boat.

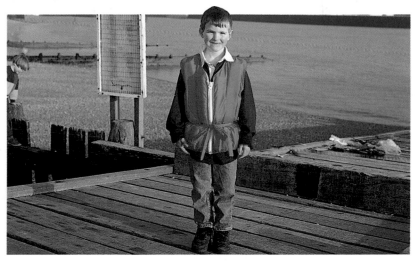

Water can be dangerous,
even if you know how
to swim.

25

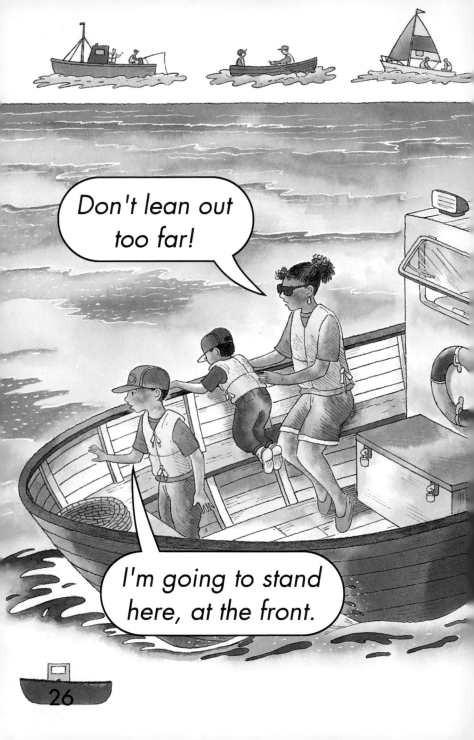

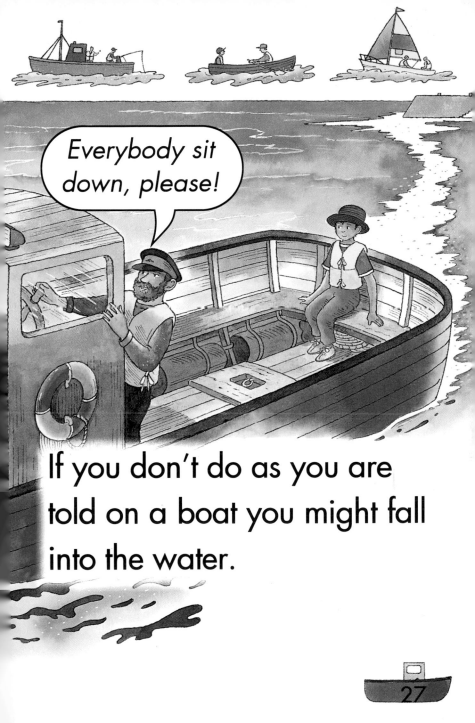

If you don't do as you are told on a boat you might fall into the water.

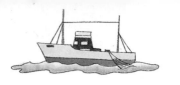
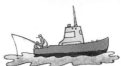
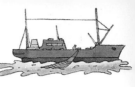
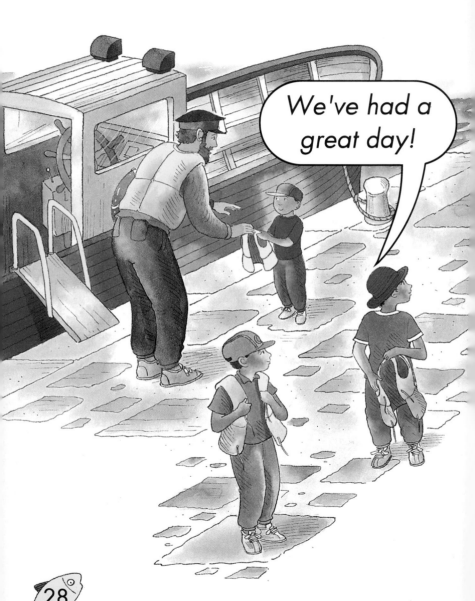

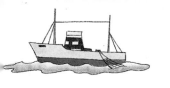
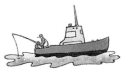
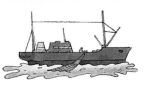

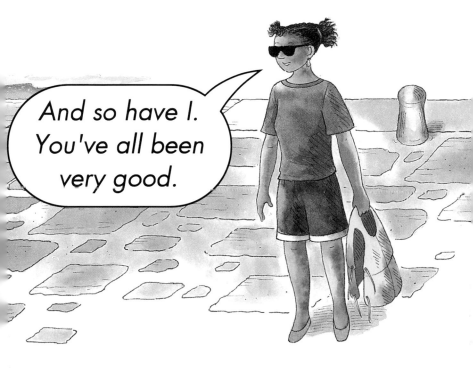

Always be sensible when you are near water and you'll have lots of fun.

Some of these children are being sensible near water and some are being silly. Do you know which are which?

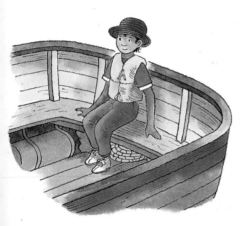

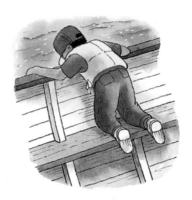

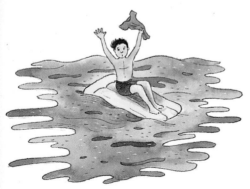

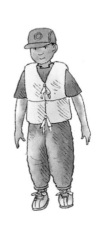